THE VEGETARIAN COOKBOOK

The Ultimate Guide to Easy & Delicious High Protein, Low Carb Vegetarian Recipes for Weight Loss and Healthy Living

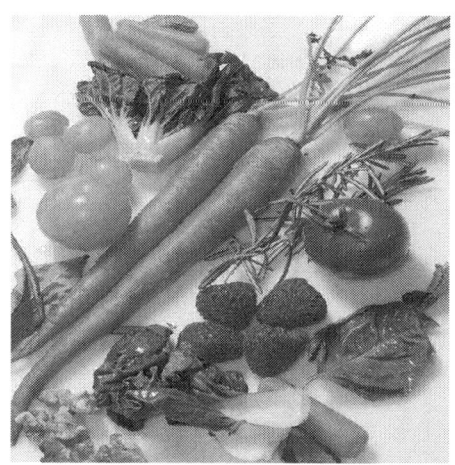

SUSAN VICTORIA

Copyright © [2023] by [Susan Victoria]

All rights reserved. No part of this publication may be reproduced, distributed, or transmitted in any form or by any means, including photocopying, recording, or other electronic or mechanical methods, without the prior written permission of the publisher, except in the case of brief quotations embodied in critical reviews and certain other noncommercial uses permitted by copyright law

TABLE OF CONTENT

INTRODUCTION 7

CHAPTER ONE 11

   Benefits of Vegetarian 1200 Calorie Diet 13

   The Importance of Calorie Counting 16

   Building a Balanced Meal 20

CHAPTER TWO 23

   21-Day Meal Plan: 23

   Week 1 23

   Week 2 26

   Week 3 and Week 4 28

CHAPTER THREE 29

   BREAKFAST DELIGHTS 29

   Energizing Smoothie Bowls: 29

   Wholesome Oatmeal Variations: 30

   Protein-Packed Breakfast Burritos: 31

   Fluffy Pancakes with Fruit Compote: 33

   Nutritious Avocado Toast Combinations: 35

CHAPTER FOUR 36

   SATISFYING SOUPS AND SALADS 36

Hearty Lentil and Vegetable Soup 36

Creamy Tomato Basil Soup 38

Fresh and Vibrant Greek Salad: 40

Roasted Vegetable Quinoa Salad: 41

Spicy Chickpea Salad with Lime Dressing: 43

CHAPTER FIVE 45

NOURISHING MAIN DISHES 45

Stuffed Bell Peppers with Quinoa and Black Beans 45

Lentil and Vegetable Curry 47

Mushroom and Spinach Lasagna Rolls: 49

Vegan Sweet Potato and Black Bean Enchiladas: 51

Tofu Stir-Fry with Ginger and Garlic: 53

CHAPTER SIX 55

WHOLESOME SIDES AND SNACKS 55

Baked Zucchini Fries with Yogurt Dip 55

Crispy Baked Sweet Potato Wedges: 57

Quinoa Stuffed Mushrooms 58

Spicy Roasted Chickpeas 60

Fresh Veggie Sticks with Hummus: 61

CHAPTER SEVEN 62

DECADENT DESSERTS 63

Chocolate Avocado Mousse 63

Berry Chia Seed Pudding: 64

Vegan Banana Bread 65

Apple Cinnamon Crumble: 67

Almond Butter Energy Balls 69

CONCLUSION 72

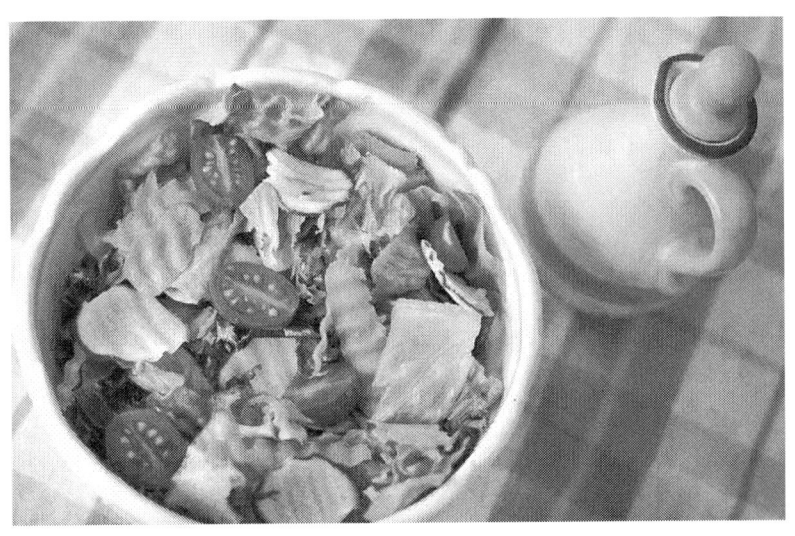

INTRODUCTION

Welcome to the world of vegetarian cuisine! In this captivating cookbook, we invite you to embark on a culinary journey that combines the principles of a vegetarian lifestyle with the goal of maintaining a balanced 1200-calorie intake. Prepare to indulge your taste buds in a symphony of flavors, all while nourishing your body and achieving your wellness goals.

Choosing a vegetarian lifestyle has become a popular choice for those seeking to embrace a healthier way of living. Whether you are a committed vegetarian or simply looking to incorporate more plant-based meals into your diet, this cookbook will be your trusted companion on your journey to optimal well-being. By focusing on nutritious, delicious, and satisfying recipes, we aim to prove that vegetarian meals can be both nourishing and satisfying, without compromising on taste.

One of the key benefits of following a vegetarian diet is its potential to support weight management and overall health. By emphasizing fresh produce, whole grains, legumes, and plant-based proteins, our recipes will help you meet your nutritional needs while keeping your caloric intake in check. Each recipe in this book has been meticulously crafted to provide a balance of macronutrients and essential vitamins and minerals, ensuring you receive the nourishment your body deserves.

Within the pages of this cookbook, you will find a treasure trove of delectable recipes that cover a wide range of culinary delights. From energizing smoothie bowls and protein-packed breakfast burritos to hearty soups, vibrant salads, comforting main courses, and delightful desserts, we have curated a diverse collection that will suit your tastes and satisfy your cravings. Each recipe is accompanied by a detailed list of ingredients, step-by-step instructions, and approximate caloric counts, allowing you to easily track your daily intake.

In addition to the 1200-calorie meal plan, we also provide the flexibility to mix and match recipes to create your own personalized menu. We understand that everyone's dietary needs and preferences are unique, so we encourage you to tailor your meal plan to suit your individual goals and lifestyle. With a wide array of recipes at your fingertips, you can effortlessly create a well-rounded and satisfying meal plan that works for you.

Prepare to be inspired as you explore the mouthwatering possibilities that await you in this Vegetarian 1200 Calorie Cookbook.

Say goodbye to bland and uninspiring meals, and say hello to a world of flavors, textures, and wholesome ingredients that will transform the way you approach vegetarian cooking. Get ready to embark on a culinary adventure that nourishes your body, delights your palate, and sets you on a path to a healthier and more vibrant you.

So, tie on your apron, sharpen your knives, and let the vegetarian feast begin!

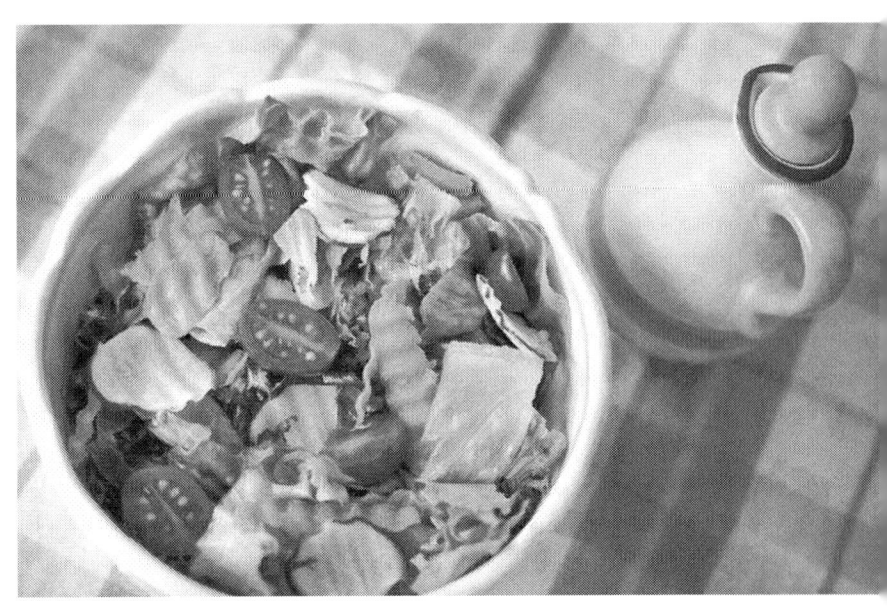

CHAPTER ONE

A vegetarian diet is not only a personal choice but also one that offers numerous benefits for both your health and the environment. In this section, we will explore the advantages of adopting a vegetarian lifestyle.

First and foremost, a vegetarian diet is rich in plant-based foods such as fruits, vegetables, legumes, whole grains, nuts, and seeds. These foods are packed with essential vitamins, minerals, and antioxidants that support overall well-being. Research has shown that vegetarians tend to have lower risks of developing chronic diseases, including heart disease, high blood pressure, obesity, and certain types of cancer.

Additionally, a vegetarian diet is typically lower in saturated fats and cholesterol found in animal-based products. This can contribute to healthier cholesterol levels, reducing the risk of cardiovascular problems. Vegetarians also tend to have lower body mass indexes (BMIs) and lower rates of obesity, which can lead to better weight management and improved metabolic health.

From an environmental standpoint, adopting a vegetarian diet can significantly reduce your carbon footprint. Livestock farming is a major contributor to greenhouse gas emissions, deforestation, and water pollution. By choosing plant-based alternatives, you are supporting sustainable agriculture and reducing the strain on natural resources, making a positive impact on the planet.

Benefits of Vegetarian 1200 Calorie Diet

The Vegetarian 1200 Calorie Diet combines the benefits of a vegetarian lifestyle with the advantages of calorie control. By following this specific approach, individuals can experience a range of benefits that contribute to their overall health and well-being. Let's explore the significant benefits of the Vegetarian 1200 Calorie Diet:

1. Effective Weight Management: The 1200 calorie limit of this diet provides a structured approach to calorie control, making it easier to achieve and maintain a healthy weight. By consuming a controlled number of calories, individuals can create a calorie deficit, which is essential for weight loss. Vegetarian meals, rich in plant-based proteins, fiber, and whole grains, contribute to satiety and can help curb overeating, making weight management more attainable.

2. Balanced Nutrient Intake: The Vegetarian 1200 Calorie Diet emphasizes the consumption of nutrient-dense foods, including fruits, vegetables, legumes, whole grains, nuts, and seeds. These plant-based ingredients offer a wide range of essential vitamins, minerals, antioxidants, and phytochemicals. By focusing on nutrient-rich foods, individuals can ensure that their bodies receive the necessary nourishment while adhering to the calorie limit.

3. Heart-Healthy Benefits: The Vegetarian 1200 Calorie Diet, by its nature, includes foods that are beneficial for heart health. By avoiding animal products, individuals reduce their intake of saturated fats and cholesterol, both of which can contribute to heart disease. Plant-based sources of protein, such as legumes and tofu, along with heart-healthy fats from sources like avocados and nuts, further promote cardiovascular well-being.

4. Lower Risk of Chronic Diseases: Numerous studies have shown that a vegetarian diet, when properly balanced, can lower the risk of chronic diseases such as type 2 diabetes, certain types of cancer, and hypertension. The Vegetarian 1200 Calorie Diet, with its focus on whole foods and controlled calorie intake, provides an opportunity to optimize nutrient intake and reduce the risk of developing these conditions.

5. Increased Fiber Intake: The diet's emphasis on fruits, vegetables, whole grains, and legumes naturally increases fiber consumption. Adequate fiber intake has several benefits, including improved digestion, better blood sugar control, and enhanced weight management. Fiber-rich foods promote satiety and can help individuals feel fuller for longer periods, reducing the likelihood of overeating and supporting weight loss efforts.

6. Sustainable and Environmentally Friendly: The Vegetarian 1200 Calorie Diet aligns with sustainable and eco-friendly practices. By reducing reliance on animal agriculture, individuals contribute to reducing greenhouse gas emissions, land degradation, and water pollution. Choosing plant-based alternatives for protein and incorporating a variety of plant foods helps promote a more sustainable and environmentally conscious approach to eating.

7. Versatility and Culinary Exploration: Following a Vegetarian 1200 Calorie Diet opens up a world of culinary possibilities. It encourages individuals to explore a diverse range of plant-based ingredients, experiment with new recipes, and develop cooking skills. With a focus on nutrient-dense, flavorful meals, individuals can enjoy a variety of delicious vegetarian dishes while still adhering to the calorie limit.

The Importance of Calorie Counting

Calorie counting plays a crucial role in weight management, promoting awareness of energy intake, and helping individuals make informed decisions about their dietary choices. Understanding the importance of calorie counting can empower individuals to achieve their health and weight goals effectively. Here are several reasons why calorie counting is significant:

- **Creating a Caloric Balance**: Calorie counting allows individuals to establish a balance between the calories consumed and the calories expended. To maintain a stable weight, it is important to consume approximately the same number of calories as the body burns. By tracking and controlling calorie intake, individuals can adjust their eating habits to achieve this balance, whether their goal is weight loss, maintenance, or even weight gain.
- **Weight Management**: Calorie counting is an effective tool for weight management. To lose weight, it is necessary to create a calorie deficit by consuming fewer calories than the body requires.

Conversely, to gain weight, a calorie surplus is needed. By understanding the specific calorie needs of their bodies, individuals can tailor their eating patterns to achieve their desired weight goals.

- **Awareness of Food Choices**: Calorie counting fosters awareness of the energy content of different foods. It provides insight into the caloric value of specific ingredients, portion sizes, and food combinations. This awareness allows individuals to make more informed choices about their meals and snacks, enabling them to opt for lower-calorie options or adjust portion sizes to align with their calorie targets.
- **Portion Con**trol: Calorie counting helps individuals develop a better understanding of appropriate portion sizes. It can be easy to underestimate the caloric content of certain foods, leading to unintentional overeating. By tracking calories, individuals can identify appropriate portion sizes and adjust their servings accordingly. This practice promotes better portion control and supports weight management efforts.

- **Identifying Hidden Calor**ies: Many foods and beverages contain hidden calories that may not be immediately apparent. Calorie counting helps uncover these hidden sources of energy, such as sugary drinks, dressings, sauces, and snacks. By accounting for these hidden calories, individuals can make conscious choices to reduce or eliminate them from their diets, thereby optimizing their calorie intake.
- **Personal Accountability**: Calorie counting holds individuals accountable for their dietary choices. It provides a tangible way to monitor progress and adherence to specific calorie goals. This accountability can serve as a source of motivation and discipline, as individuals take ownership of their eating habits and strive to meet their calorie targets.
- **Individualized Approac**h: Every person has unique calorie requirements based on factors such as age, gender, weight, height, and activity level. Calorie counting allows individuals to personalize their approach to nutrition based on their specific needs. It helps them determine the optimal calorie intake for their goals, ensuring that they are

providing their bodies with adequate nourishment while still adhering to their desired calorie range.

Overall, calorie counting is a valuable tool for weight management, promoting awareness of food choices, portion control, and personal accountability. By incorporating calorie counting into their lifestyle, individuals can make more informed decisions about their dietary intake, optimize their calorie balance, and work towards achieving their health and weight goals.

Building a Balanced Meal

Building a balanced meal is essential for ensuring optimal nutrition and supporting overall health and well-being. A well-rounded, balanced meal should include a combination of macronutrients (carbohydrates, proteins, and fats), as well as an array of micronutrients (vitamins and minerals). Here are some key considerations and guidelines for building a balanced meal:

1. **Include a Source of Protein**: Protein is essential for tissue repair, muscle growth, and numerous other physiological functions. Incorporate a lean protein source into your meal, such as tofu, tempeh, legumes, lentils, beans, quinoa, or Greek yogurt. These options provide high-quality protein while also offering other nutrients like fiber and minerals.

2. **Choose Complex Carbohydrates**: Carbohydrates are a vital energy source for the body. Opt for complex carbohydrates that provide sustained energy and are rich in fiber, such as whole grains (oats, brown rice, quinoa), whole-wheat products, sweet potatoes, and legumes. These carbohydrates

are digested more slowly, preventing blood sugar spikes and promoting satiety.

3. **Include a Variety of Colorful Vegetables:** Vegetables are packed with essential vitamins, minerals, and fiber. Aim to fill half of your plate with a variety of colorful vegetables, including leafy greens, broccoli, bell peppers, carrots, tomatoes, and cucumbers. These nutrient-dense foods provide antioxidants that support overall health and protect against chronic diseases.

4. **Incorporate Healthy Fats:** Include a moderate amount of healthy fats in your meals, as they are necessary for nutrient absorption and provide satiety. Opt for sources like avocados, nuts, seeds, olive oil, and fatty fish (if pescatarian). These fats contain omega-3 fatty acids and monounsaturated fats, which support heart health and cognitive function.

5. **Don't Forget About Fiber:** Fiber is crucial for digestive health, maintaining a healthy weight, and preventing chronic diseases. Ensure your meal includes a good source of fiber, such as whole grains, legumes, fruits, and vegetables. High-fiber

foods promote satiety and help regulate blood sugar levels.

6. **Mindful Portion Control**: Pay attention to portion sizes to avoid overeating and maintain a calorie balance. Use visual cues, such as dividing your plate into sections, to ensure you have appropriate portions of each food group. Practice mindful eating, savoring each bite and eating slowly to recognize when you feel comfortably full.
7. **Hydrate with Water**: Don't forget to hydrate! Water is essential for overall health and helps with digestion, nutrient absorption, and regulating body temperature. Drink water with your meal, and limit sugary beverages and excessive alcohol consumption.

Remember, everyone's nutritional needs may vary based on factors such as age, gender, activity level, and specific dietary requirements.

A sample Dietary Plan is presented in the next chapter, feel free to experiment with different arrangements as long it is still within the required 1200 daily calorie.

CHAPTER TWO

21-Day Meal Plan:

Week 1:

Day 1:

Breakfast: Energizing Smoothie Bowl

Lunch: Hearty Lentil and Vegetable Soup

Dinner: Stuffed Bell Peppers with Quinoa and Black Beans

Snacks: Fresh Veggie Sticks with Hummus, Almond Butter Energy Balls

Day 2:

Breakfast: Wholesome Oatmeal with Fruit Toppings

Lunch: Creamy Tomato Basil Soup

Dinner: Lentil and Vegetable Curry

Snacks: Spicy Roasted Chickpeas, Berry Chia Seed Pudding

Day 3:

Breakfast: Protein-Packed Breakfast Burritos

Lunch: Fresh and Vibrant Greek Salad

Dinner: Mushroom and Spinach Lasagna Rolls

Snacks: Baked Zucchini Fries with Yogurt Dip, Apple Cinnamon Crumble

Day 4:

Breakfast: Fluffy Pancakes with Fruit Compote

Lunch: Roasted Vegetable Quinoa Salad

Dinner: Vegan Sweet Potato and Black Bean Enchiladas

Snacks: Quinoa Stuffed Mushrooms, Chocolate Avocado Mousse

Day 5:

Breakfast: Nutritious Avocado Toast with Various Toppings

Lunch: Spicy Chickpea Salad with Lime Dressing

Dinner: Tofu Stir-Fry with Ginger and Garlic

Snacks: Crispy Baked Sweet Potato Wedges, Vegan Banana Bread

Day 6:

Breakfast: Energizing Smoothie Bowl

Lunch: Hearty Lentil and Vegetable Soup

Dinner: Stuffed Bell Peppers with Quinoa and Black Beans

Snacks: Fresh Veggie Sticks with Hummus, Almond Butter Energy Balls

Day 7:

Breakfast: Wholesome Oatmeal with Fruit Toppings

Lunch: Creamy Tomato Basil Soup

Dinner: Lentil and Vegetable Curry

Snacks: Spicy Roasted Chickpeas, Berry Chia Seed Pudding

Week 2
Day 1:

Breakfast: Nutritious Avocado Toast with Various Toppings
Lunch: Spicy Chickpea Salad with Lime Dressing
Dinner: Tofu Stir-Fry with Ginger and Garlic
Snacks: Crispy Baked Sweet Potato Wedges, Vegan Banana Bread

Day 2:

Breakfast: Energizing Smoothie Bowl

Lunch: Hearty Lentil and Vegetable Soup

Dinner: Stuffed Bell Peppers with Quinoa and Black Beans

Snacks: Fresh Veggie Sticks with Hummus, Almond Butter Energy Balls

Day 3:

Breakfast: Wholesome Oatmeal with Fruit Toppings

Lunch: Creamy Tomato Basil Soup

Dinner: Lentil and Vegetable Curry

Snacks: Spicy Roasted Chickpeas, Berry Chia Seed

Day 4:

Breakfast: Energizing Smoothie Bowl

Lunch: Hearty Lentil and Vegetable Soup

Dinner: Stuffed Bell Peppers with Quinoa and Black Beans

Snacks: Fresh Veggie Sticks with Hummus, Almond Butter Energy Balls

Day 5:

Breakfast: Wholesome Oatmeal with Fruit Toppings

Lunch: Creamy Tomato Basil Soup

Dinner: Lentil and Vegetable Curry

Snacks: Spicy Roasted Chickpeas, Berry Chia Seed Pudding

Day 6:

Breakfast: Protein-Packed Breakfast Burritos

Lunch: Fresh and Vibrant Greek Salad

Dinner: Mushroom and Spinach Lasagna Rolls

Snacks: Baked Zucchini Fries with Yogurt Dip, Apple Cinnamon Crumble

Day 7:

Breakfast: Fluffy Pancakes with Fruit Compote

Lunch: Roasted Vegetable Quinoa Salad

Dinner: Vegan Sweet Potato and Black Bean Enchiladas

Snacks: Quinoa Stuffed Mushrooms, Chocolate Avocado Mousse

Pudding

Week 3 and Week 4

REPEAT the meal plan from Weeks 1 and 2

Feel free to experiment with different arrangements as long it is still within the required 1200 daily calorie.

Remember to adjust the recipes and portion sizes based on your dietary needs and preferences.

Enjoy your vegetarian culinary journey!

CHAPTER THREE

BREAKFAST DELIGHTS

Energizing Smoothie Bowls:

Ingredients:
- 1 ripe banana
- 1 cup frozen berries (such as strawberries, blueberries, or mixed berries)
- 1/2 cup plain Greek yogurt
- 1/4 cup almond milk (or any plant-based milk)
- Toppings: sliced fresh fruits, granola, nuts, seeds, coconut flakes, etc.

Method of Preparation:

1. In a blender, combine the ripe banana, frozen berries, Greek yogurt, and almond milk.
2. Blend until smooth and creamy.
3. Pour the smoothie mixture into a bowl.
4. Top with your favorite toppings, such as sliced fresh fruits, granola, nuts, seeds, and coconut flakes.
5. Enjoy with a spoon!

Number of Servings: 1

Approximate Caloric Count: Around 300-400 calories per serving (depending on the choice and amount of toppings)

Average Preparation Time: 5 minutes

Wholesome Oatmeal Variations:
Ingredients:

- 1/2 cup rolled oats

- 1 cup water or milk (dairy or plant-based)

- Optional toppings: fresh or dried fruits, nuts, seeds, honey, maple syrup, cinnamon, etc.

Method of Preparation:

1. In a saucepan, bring the water or milk to a boil.
2. Add the rolled oats and reduce the heat to low.
3. Cook the oats for about 5 minutes, stirring occasionally, until they reach your desired consistency.
4. Remove from heat and let it sit for a minute.
5. Transfer the cooked oats to a bowl.
6. Add your preferred toppings, such as fresh or dried fruits, nuts, seeds, honey, maple syrup, or cinnamon.
7. Stir well and enjoy!

Number of Servings: 1

Approximate Caloric Count: Around 150-250 calories per serving (depending on the choice and amount of toppings)

Average Preparation Time: 10-15 minutes

Protein-Packed Breakfast Burritos:

Ingredients:

- 2 large whole wheat tortillas
- 4 large eggs, beaten
- 1/4 cup diced bell peppers
- 1/4 cup diced onions
- 1/4 cup diced tomatoes
- 1/4 cup shredded cheese (such as cheddar or Mexican blend)
- Salt and pepper to taste
- Optional toppings: avocado, salsa, sour cream, etc.

Method of Preparation:

1. In a skillet, heat a small amount of oil over medium heat.
2. Add the diced bell peppers, onions, and tomatoes to the skillet and sauté until softened.
3. Pour the beaten eggs into the skillet and scramble them with the vegetables until fully cooked.
4. Season with salt and pepper to taste.
5. Warm the tortillas in a separate skillet or in the microwave.
6. Divide the scrambled eggs and vegetable mixture between the tortillas.
7. Sprinkle shredded cheese on top.
8. Roll up the tortillas, tucking in the sides to create a burrito shape.

9. Optional: You can lightly grill the burritos in a skillet to melt the cheese and make them crispy.
10. Serve with optional toppings like avocado, salsa, or sour cream.

Number of Servings: 2

Approximate Caloric Count: Around 350-400 calories per serving (depending on the choice and amount of toppings)

Average Preparation Time: 15-20 minutes

Fluffy Pancakes with Fruit Compote:

Ingredients:

- 1 cup all-purpose flour

- 1 tablespoon sugar

- 1 teaspoon baking powder

- 1/2 teaspoon baking soda

- 1/4 teaspoon salt

- 1 cup buttermilk (or 1 cup milk mixed with 1 tablespoon lemon juice or vinegar)

- 1 large egg

- 1 tablespoon melted butter

- Fruit Compote: mixed berries (fresh or frozen), sugar, water

Method of Preparation:

1. In a mixing bowl, whisk together the flour, sugar, baking powder, baking soda, and salt.
2. In a separate bowl, whisk together the buttermilk, egg, and melted butter.
3. Pour the wet ingredients into the dry ingredients and stir until just combined (some lumps are okay).
4. Let the batter rest for a few minutes.

5. Preheat a non-stick skillet or griddle over medium heat.
6. Pour 1/4 cup of batter onto the skillet for each pancake.
7. Cook until bubbles form on the surface, then flip and cook the other side until golden brown.
8. Repeat with the remaining batter.
9. For the fruit compote, in a small saucepan, combine the mixed berries, sugar, and a splash of water.
10. Simmer the mixture over low heat, stirring occasionally until the berries break down and the sauce thickens slightly.
11. Serve the fluffy pancakes with the warm fruit compote on top.

Number of Servings: 2-3 (depending on the size of the pancakes)

Approximate Caloric Count: Around 200-250 calories per serving (excluding fruit compote)

Average Preparation Time: 20-30 minutes

Nutritious Avocado Toast Combinations:

Ingredients:
- 2 slices of whole grain bread
- 1 ripe avocado
- Salt and pepper to taste
- Optional toppings: sliced tomatoes, cucumber, radish, sprouts, feta cheese, red pepper flakes, etc.

Method of Preparation:

1. Toast the bread slices to your desired level of crispness.
2. Cut the ripe avocado in half, remove the pit, and scoop out the flesh into a bowl.
3. Mash the avocado with a fork until it reaches your preferred consistency (smooth or chunky).
4. Season the mashed avocado with salt and pepper to taste.
5. Spread the mashed avocado evenly onto the toasted bread slices.
6. Add your favorite toppings, such as sliced tomatoes, cucumber, radish, sprouts, feta cheese, or a sprinkle of red pepper flakes.
7. Serve the avocado toast immediately.

Number of Servings: 1-2 (depending on the size of the avocado and bread slices)

Approximate Caloric Count: Around 250-350 calories per serving (depending on the type and amount of toppings)

Average Preparation Time: 5-10 minutes

CHAPTER FOUR

SATISFYING SOUPS AND SALADS
Hearty Lentil and Vegetable Soup:

Ingredients:
- 1 cup dried green or brown lentils, rinsed
- 1 tablespoon olive oil
- 1 onion, diced
- 2 carrots, diced
- 2 celery stalks, diced
- 2 cloves garlic, minced
- 1 teaspoon ground cumin
- 1 teaspoon ground coriander
- 1 teaspoon dried thyme
- 4 cups vegetable broth
- 2 cups water
- Salt and pepper to taste
- Fresh parsley, chopped (for garnish)

Method of Preparation:

1. In a large pot, heat the olive oil over medium heat.
2. Add the diced onion, carrots, celery, and minced garlic. Sauté until the vegetables are softened.
3. Add the ground cumin, ground coriander, and dried thyme. Stir to coat the vegetables with the spices.
4. Add the rinsed lentils, vegetable broth, and water to the pot.

5. Bring the soup to a boil, then reduce the heat and simmer for about 25-30 minutes, or until the lentils are tender.
6. Season with salt and pepper to taste.
7. Serve hot, garnished with fresh parsley.

Number of Servings: 4-6

Approximate Caloric Count: Around 200-250 calories per serving

Average Preparation Time: 45 minutes

Creamy Tomato Basil Soup:

Ingredients:

- 1 tablespoon olive oil
- 1 onion, diced
- 2 cloves garlic, minced
- 1 can (14 ounces) diced tomatoes
- 2 cups vegetable broth
- 1/2 cup unsweetened coconut milk (or heavy cream for a non-vegan option)
- 1/4 cup fresh basil leaves, chopped
- Salt and pepper to taste

Method of Preparation:

1. In a large pot, heat the olive oil over medium heat.
2. Add the diced onion and minced garlic. Sauté until the onion becomes translucent.
3. Add the diced tomatoes (including the juice) to the pot and stir well.
4. Pour in the vegetable broth and bring the mixture to a boil.
5. Reduce the heat and simmer for about 15-20 minutes to allow the flavors to blend together.
6. Remove the pot from heat and let it cool slightly.

7. Using an immersion blender or regular blender, puree the soup until smooth.
8. Return the soup to the pot and stir in the coconut milk (or heavy cream) and chopped basil.
9. Season with salt and pepper to taste.
10. Reheat the soup gently before serving.

Number of Servings: 4-6

Approximate Caloric Count: Around 150-200 calories per serving

Average Preparation Time: 30-40 minutes

Fresh and Vibrant Greek Salad:

Ingredients:
- 2 large cucumbers, diced
- 4 Roma tomatoes, diced
- 1 red onion, thinly sliced
- 1 bell pepper (green, red, or yellow), diced
- 1 cup Kalamata olives, pitted and halved
- 1 cup crumbled feta cheese
- 1/4 cup fresh parsley, chopped
- 1/4 cup extra virgin olive oil
- 2 tablespoons red wine vinegar
- Salt and pepper to taste

Method of Preparation:

1. In a large bowl, combine the diced cucumbers, tomatoes, red onion, bell pepper, Kalamata olives, crumbled feta cheese, and fresh parsley.
2. In a separate small bowl, whisk together the extra virgin olive oil, red wine vinegar, salt, and pepper to make the dressing.
3. Pour the dressing over the salad ingredients and toss gently to coat everything evenly.
4. Adjust the seasoning if needed.
5. Let the salad sit for about 10-15 minutes to allow the flavors to meld together.
6. Serve chilled as a refreshing side dish.

Number of Servings: 4-6

Approximate Caloric Count: Around 200-250 calories per serving

Average Preparation Time: 15-20 minutes

Roasted Vegetable Quinoa Salad:

Ingredients:

- 1 cup quinoa
- 2 cups water or vegetable broth
- 2 cups mixed vegetables (such as bell peppers, zucchini, eggplant, cherry tomatoes, etc.), cut into bite-sized pieces
- 2 tablespoons olive oil
- 2 cloves garlic, minced
- 1 teaspoon dried herbs (such as thyme, rosemary, or Italian seasoning)
- Salt and pepper to taste
- Juice of 1 lemon
- Fresh parsley or basil, chopped (for garnish)

Method of Preparation:

1. Rinse the quinoa under cold water.
2. In a saucepan, bring the water or vegetable broth to a boil.
3. Add the rinsed quinoa and reduce the heat to low.
4. Cover and simmer for about 15-20 minutes, or until the quinoa is cooked and the liquid is absorbed.
5. Meanwhile, preheat the oven to 400°F (200°C).
6. In a large bowl, toss the mixed vegetables with olive oil, minced garlic, dried herbs, salt, and pepper until evenly coated.
7. Spread the vegetables on a baking sheet in a single layer.

8. Roast in the preheated oven for about 20-25 minutes, or until the vegetables are tender and slightly caramelized.
9. In a large serving bowl, combine the cooked quinoa and roasted vegetables.
10. Squeeze the lemon juice over the salad and toss gently to combine.
11. Garnish with fresh parsley or basil before serving.

Number of Servings: 4-6

Approximate Caloric Count: Around 250-300 calories per serving

Average Preparation Time: 40-50 minutes

Spicy Chickpea Salad with Lime Dressing:

Ingredients:

- 2 cans (15 ounces each) chickpeas (garbanzo beans), drained and rinsed
- 1 cup cherry tomatoes, halved
- 1 cucumber, diced
- 1 bell pepper (any color), diced
- 1 small red onion, finely chopped
- 1 jalapeño pepper, seeds removed and finely chopped
- 1/4 cup fresh cilantro, chopped
- Juice of 2 limes
- 2 tablespoons olive oil
- 1 teaspoon ground cumin
- 1/2 teaspoon chili powder (adjust according to spice preference)
- Salt and pepper to taste

Method of Preparation:

1. In a large bowl, combine the drained and rinsed chickpeas, cherry tomatoes, cucumber, bell pepper, red onion, jalapeño pepper, and fresh cilantro.
2. In a small bowl, whisk together the lime juice, olive oil, ground cumin, chili powder, salt, and pepper to make the dressing.

3. Pour the dressing over the chickpea salad and toss well to coat everything evenly.
4. Adjust the seasoning if needed.
5. Let the salad marinate in the refrigerator for about 30 minutes to allow the flavors to meld together.
6. Serve chilled as a zesty and flavorful salad.

Number of Servings: 4-6

Approximate Caloric Count: Around 200-250 calories per serving

Average Preparation Time: 20-30 minutes

CHAPTER FIVE

NOURISHING MAIN DISHES

Stuffed Bell Peppers with Quinoa and Black Beans:

Ingredients:
- 4 bell peppers (any color)
- 1 cup cooked quinoa
- 1 cup black beans, drained and rinsed
- 1 cup corn kernels (fresh or frozen)
- 1/2 cup diced tomatoes
- 1/2 cup shredded cheese (such as cheddar or Monterey Jack)
- 1/4 cup chopped fresh cilantro
- 1 teaspoon cumin
- 1 teaspoon chili powder
- Salt and pepper to taste
- Optional toppings: sliced avocado, sour cream, salsa

Method of Preparation:

1. Preheat the oven to 375°F (190°C).
2. Slice off the tops of the bell peppers and remove the seeds and membranes.
3. In a mixing bowl, combine the cooked quinoa, black beans, corn kernels, diced tomatoes, shredded

cheese, chopped cilantro, cumin, chili powder, salt, and pepper.
4. Stuff the mixture evenly into the bell peppers.
5. Place the stuffed bell peppers in a baking dish and cover with foil.
6. Bake in the preheated oven for about 25-30 minutes, or until the bell peppers are tender and the filling is heated through.
7. Remove from the oven and let them cool slightly.
8. Serve the stuffed bell peppers with optional toppings such as sliced avocado, sour cream, or salsa.

Number of Servings: 4

Approximate Caloric Count: Around 300-350 calories per serving

Average Preparation Time: 45-60 minutes

Lentil and Vegetable Curry:

Ingredients:

- 1 cup dried lentils (green or brown), rinsed
- 1 tablespoon olive oil
- 1 onion, diced
- 2 cloves garlic, minced
- 1 bell pepper (any color), diced
- 2 carrots, diced
- 1 zucchini, diced
- 1 can (14 ounces) diced tomatoes
- 1 can (14 ounces) coconut milk
- 2 tablespoons curry powder
- 1 teaspoon ground cumin
- 1 teaspoon ground coriander
- Salt and pepper to taste
- Fresh cilantro, chopped (for garnish)
- Cooked rice or naan bread (for serving)

Method of Preparation:

1. In a saucepan, bring 2 cups of water to a boil.
2. Add the rinsed lentils and simmer for about 15-20 minutes, or until the lentils are tender. Drain and set aside.
3. In a large pot, heat the olive oil over medium heat.
4. Add the diced onion and minced garlic. Sauté until the onion becomes translucent.
5. Add the diced bell pepper, carrots, and zucchini. Cook for a few minutes until the vegetables start to soften.

6. Stir in the diced tomatoes, coconut milk, curry powder, ground cumin, ground coriander, salt, and pepper.
7. Bring the mixture to a boil, then reduce the heat and simmer for about 15-20 minutes, or until the vegetables are tender.
8. Stir in the cooked lentils and simmer for an additional 5 minutes to heat everything through.
9. Adjust the seasoning if needed.
10. Serve the lentil and vegetable curry hot, garnished with fresh cilantro. Accompany it with cooked rice or naan bread.

Number of Servings: 4-6

Approximate Caloric Count: Around 300-350 calories per serving (excluding rice or naan bread)

Average Preparation Time: 45-60 minutes

Mushroom and Spinach Lasagna Rolls:

Ingredients:
- 8 lasagna noodles
- 2 tablespoons olive oil
- 1 onion, diced
- 2 cloves garlic, minced
- 8 ounces mushrooms, sliced
- 4 cups fresh spinach
- 1 cup ricotta cheese (or vegan ricotta substitute)
- 1/2 cup grated Parmesan cheese (or vegan Parmesan substitute)
- 1/4 cup chopped fresh basil
- 1 can (14 ounces) diced tomatoes
- 1 cup marinara sauce
- Salt and pepper to taste
- Shredded mozzarella cheese (or vegan mozzarella substitute) for topping (optional)

Method of Preparation:

1. Preheat the oven to 375°F (190°C).
2. Cook the lasagna noodles according to the package instructions until al dente. Drain and set aside.
3. In a large skillet, heat the olive oil over medium heat.
4. Add the diced onion and minced garlic. Sauté until the onion becomes translucent.
5. Add the sliced mushrooms and cook until they release their moisture and start to brown.
6. Stir in the fresh spinach and cook until wilted.

7. In a mixing bowl, combine the ricotta cheese, grated Parmesan cheese, chopped basil, salt, and pepper.
8. Spread about 1/4 cup of the ricotta mixture onto each lasagna noodle.
9. Divide the mushroom and spinach mixture evenly among the noodles, spreading it over the ricotta layer.
10. Roll up each noodle tightly and place them seam-side down in a baking dish.
11. In a separate bowl, mix together the diced tomatoes and marinara sauce. Season with salt and pepper to taste.
12. Pour the tomato sauce mixture over the lasagna rolls in the baking dish.
13. If desired, sprinkle shredded mozzarella cheese on top.
14. Cover the dish with foil and bake in the preheated oven for about 20-25 minutes, or until the rolls are heated through and the cheese is melted.
15. Remove the foil and bake for an additional 5 minutes to brown the cheese (if using).
16. Let the lasagna rolls cool slightly before serving.

Number of Servings: 4-6

Approximate Caloric Count: Around 350-400 calories per serving

Average Preparation Time: 60-75 minutes

Vegan Sweet Potato and Black Bean Enchiladas:

Ingredients:
- 2 medium sweet potatoes, peeled and diced
- 1 can (15 ounces) black beans, drained and rinsed
- 1 small onion, diced
- 2 cloves garlic, minced
- 1 teaspoon ground cumin
- 1 teaspoon chili powder
- 1/2 teaspoon smoked paprika
- Salt and pepper to taste
- 8 small tortillas (corn or flour)
- 1 cup enchilada sauce
- 1/2 cup vegan shredded cheese (such as vegan cheddar or mozzarella)
- Fresh cilantro, chopped (for garnish)
- Sliced avocado and vegan sour cream (for serving, optional)

Method of Preparation:

1. Preheat the oven to 375°F (190°C).
2. Place the diced sweet potatoes on a baking sheet and roast in the preheated oven for about 20-25 minutes, or until tender.
3. In a skillet, heat some olive oil over medium heat.
4. Add the diced onion and minced garlic. Sauté until the onion becomes translucent.
5. Add the drained black beans, ground cumin, chili powder, smoked paprika, salt, and pepper

to the skillet. Stir well to combine and cook for a few minutes.
6. In a large bowl, combine the roasted sweet potatoes and black bean mixture.
7. Warm the tortillas slightly to make them pliable.
8. Place a portion of the sweet potato and black bean filling onto each tortilla and roll it up tightly.
9. Arrange the rolled enchiladas in a baking dish, seam-side down.
10. Pour the enchilada sauce evenly over the enchiladas.
11. Sprinkle vegan shredded cheese on top.
12. Cover the dish with foil and bake in the preheated oven for about 20-25 minutes, or until the enchiladas are heated through and the cheese is melted.
13. Remove the foil and bake for an additional 5 minutes to brown the cheese.
14. Garnish with chopped cilantro before serving.
15. Serve with sliced avocado and vegan sour cream, if desired.

Number of Servings: 4-6

Approximate Caloric Count: Around 300-350 calories per serving

Average Preparation Time: 45-60 minutes

Tofu Stir-Fry with Ginger and Garlic:

Ingredients:

- 1 block (14 ounces) firm tofu, drained and cubed
- 2 tablespoons soy sauce
- 1 tablespoon cornstarch
- 2 tablespoons sesame oil
- 1 tablespoon grated fresh ginger
- 3 cloves garlic, minced
- 1 bell pepper (any color), sliced
- 1 carrot, thinly sliced
- 1 cup broccoli florets
- 1 cup snap peas
- 1 cup mushrooms, sliced
- 2 tablespoons hoisin sauce
- 1 tablespoon rice vinegar
- Salt and pepper to taste
- Cooked rice or noodles (for serving)

Method of Preparation:

1. In a bowl, combine the cubed tofu, soy sauce, and cornstarch. Toss gently to coat the tofu in the marinade. Let it sit for about 10 minutes.
2. Heat 1 tablespoon of sesame oil in a large skillet or wok over medium-high heat.
3. Add the marinated tofu cubes to the skillet and cook until golden brown on all sides. Remove the tofu from the skillet and set it aside.
4. In the same skillet, add another tablespoon of sesame oil and reduce the heat to medium.

5. Add the grated ginger and minced garlic to the skillet. Sauté for about 1 minute until fragrant.
6. Add the sliced bell pepper, carrot, broccoli florets, snap peas, and mushrooms to the skillet. Stir-fry for about 5-7 minutes, or until the vegetables are crisp-tender.
7. In a small bowl, whisk together the hoisin sauce and rice vinegar. Pour the sauce over the stir-fried vegetables.
8. Return the cooked tofu to the skillet and toss everything together to coat the tofu and vegetables in the sauce.
9. Season with salt and pepper to taste.
10. Continue cooking for another 2-3 minutes until everything is heated through.
11. Serve the tofu stir-fry hot over cooked rice or noodles.

Number of Servings: 4-6

Approximate Caloric Count: Around 250-300 calories per serving (excluding rice or noodles)

Average Preparation Time: 30-40 minutes

CHAPTER SIX

WHOLESOME SIDES AND SNACKS

Baked Zucchini Fries with Yogurt Dip:

Ingredients:
- 2 medium zucchinis
- 1/2 cup breadcrumbs
- 1/4 cup grated Parmesan cheese (or vegan Parmesan substitute)
- 1 teaspoon dried Italian seasoning
- Salt and pepper to taste
- 2 eggs (or flaxseed mixture for vegan option)
- Cooking spray
- 1 cup Greek yogurt (or vegan yogurt substitute)
- 1 tablespoon chopped fresh dill (optional)
- 1 tablespoon lemon juice
- Salt and pepper to taste

Method of Preparation:

1. Preheat the oven to 425°F (220°C).
2. Cut the zucchinis into fry-shaped strips.
3. In a shallow dish, combine the breadcrumbs, grated Parmesan cheese, dried Italian seasoning, salt, and pepper.
4. In another shallow dish, beat the eggs.

5. Dip each zucchini strip into the beaten eggs, then coat it in the breadcrumb mixture.
6. Place the coated zucchini fries on a baking sheet sprayed with cooking spray.
7. Bake in the preheated oven for about 20-25 minutes, or until the zucchini fries are golden and crispy.
8. While the fries are baking, prepare the yogurt dip by combining the Greek yogurt, chopped fresh dill (if using), lemon juice, salt, and pepper in a bowl. Mix well.
9. Serve the baked zucchini fries hot with the yogurt dip.

Number of Servings: 4

Approximate Caloric Count: Around 150-200 calories per serving

Average Preparation Time: 30-40 minutes

Crispy Baked Sweet Potato Wedges:

Ingredients:
- 2 large sweet potatoes
- 2 tablespoons olive oil
- 1 teaspoon paprika
- 1/2 teaspoon garlic powder
- 1/2 teaspoon onion powder
- 1/2 teaspoon dried thyme
- Salt and pepper to taste
- Cooking spray

Method of Preparation:

1. Preheat the oven to 425°F (220°C).
2. Scrub the sweet potatoes and cut them into wedges.
3. In a large bowl, toss the sweet potato wedges with olive oil, paprika, garlic powder, onion powder, dried thyme, salt, and pepper until well coated.
4. Place the seasoned sweet potato wedges on a baking sheet sprayed with cooking spray, making sure they are in a single layer.
5. Bake in the preheated oven for about 25-30 minutes, or until the sweet potato wedges are crispy and golden brown.
6. Serve the crispy baked sweet potato wedges hot.

Number of Servings: 4

Approximate Caloric Count: Around 150-200 calories per serving

Average Preparation Time: 35-45 minutes

Quinoa Stuffed Mushrooms:

Ingredients:
- 12 large mushrooms
- 1 cup cooked quinoa
- 1/4 cup diced onion
- 1/4 cup diced bell pepper (any color)
- 2 cloves garlic, minced
- 1/4 cup chopped fresh parsley
- 1/4 cup grated Parmesan cheese (or vegan Parmesan substitute)
- Salt and pepper to taste
- Cooking spray

Method of Preparation:

1. Preheat the oven to 375°F (190°C).
2. Remove the stems from the mushrooms and finely chop them.
3. In a skillet, heat some olive oil over medium heat.
4. Add the diced onion, diced bell pepper, minced garlic, and chopped mushroom stems to the skillet. Sauté until the vegetables are softened.
5. In a mixing bowl, combine the cooked quinoa, sautéed vegetable mixture, chopped fresh parsley, grated Parmesan cheese, salt, and pepper. Mix well.
6. Place the mushroom caps on a baking sheet sprayed with cooking spray, cavity side up.
7. Spoon the quinoa mixture into the mushroom caps, pressing it down gently.

8. Bake in the preheated oven for about 20-25 minutes, or until the mushrooms are tender and the filling is heated through.
9. Serve the quinoa stuffed mushrooms hot.

Number of Servings: 4

Approximate Caloric Count: Around 100-150 calories per serving

Average Preparation Time: 40-50 minutes

Spicy Roasted Chickpeas:

Ingredients:
- 2 cans (15 ounces each) chickpeas (garbanzo beans), drained and rinsed
- 2 tablespoons olive oil
- 1 teaspoon chili powder
- 1/2 teaspoon cumin
- 1/2 teaspoon paprika
- 1/4 teaspoon cayenne pepper (adjust to taste)
- Salt to taste

Method of Preparation:

1. Preheat the oven to 400°F (200°C).
2. Place the drained and rinsed chickpeas on a baking sheet lined with parchment paper or foil. Pat them dry with a paper towel.
3. In a small bowl, combine the olive oil, chili powder, cumin, paprika, cayenne pepper, and salt.
4. Drizzle the spice mixture over the chickpeas and toss until they are evenly coated.
5. Spread the seasoned chickpeas in a single layer on the baking sheet.
6. Roast in the preheated oven for about 25-30 minutes, or until the chickpeas are crispy and golden brown.
7. Remove from the oven and let them cool slightly before serving.

Number of Servings: 4 **Approximate Caloric Count**: Around 150-200 calories per serving

Average Preparation Time: 35-45 minutes

Fresh Veggie Sticks with Hummus:

Ingredients:

- Assorted fresh vegetables (carrots, celery, bell peppers, cucumbers, etc.), cut into sticks

- Store-bought or homemade hummus

Method of Preparation:

1. Wash and prepare the vegetables by cutting them into sticks.
2. Arrange the vegetable sticks on a platter.
3. Serve the fresh veggie sticks with hummus as a dip.

Number of Servings: 4

Approximate Caloric Count: Varies depending on the types and quantities of vegetables and hummus used

Average Preparation Time: 10-15 minutes

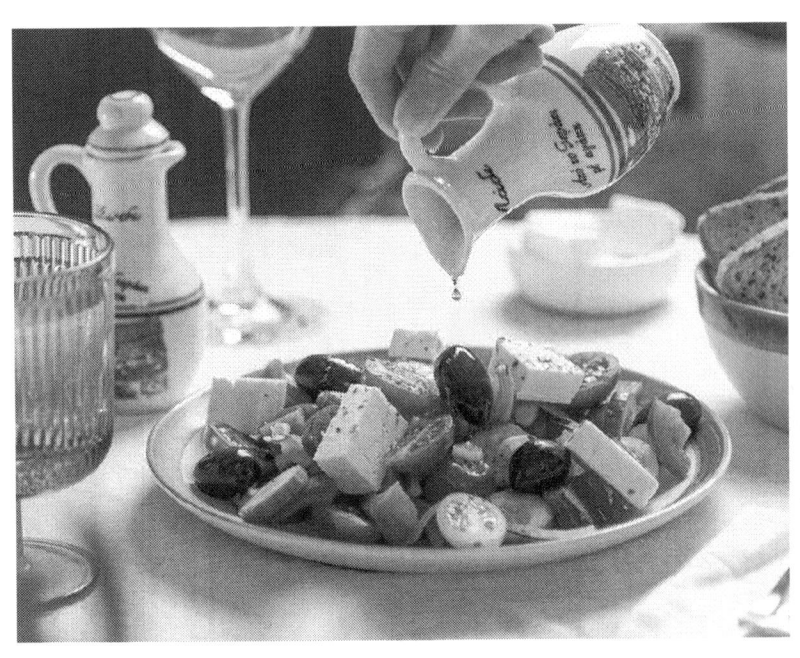

CHAPTER SEVEN

DECADENT DESSERTS

Chocolate Avocado Mousse:

Ingredients:
- 2 ripe avocados
- 1/4 cup unsweetened cocoa powder
- 1/4 cup maple syrup or agave nectar
- 1/4 cup almond milk (or any plant-based milk)
- 1 teaspoon vanilla extract
- Pinch of salt
- Optional toppings: sliced strawberries, shaved dark chocolate, chopped nuts

Method of Preparation:

1. Cut the avocados in half, remove the pits, and scoop out the flesh into a blender or food processor.
2. Add the cocoa powder, maple syrup (or agave nectar), almond milk, vanilla extract, and salt to the blender.
3. Blend until smooth and creamy, scraping down the sides as needed.
4. Taste and adjust the sweetness if desired by adding more maple syrup or agave nectar.
5. Transfer the chocolate avocado mousse to serving dishes or glasses.
6. Refrigerate for at least 1-2 hours to chill and set.
7. Before serving, garnish with sliced strawberries, shaved dark chocolate, or chopped nuts, if desired.

Number of Servings: 4 **Approximate Caloric Count**: Around 150-200 calories per serving

Berry Chia Seed Pudding:

Ingredients:
- 1/4 cup chia seeds
- 1 cup almond milk (or any plant-based milk)
- 1 tablespoon maple syrup or agave nectar
- 1/2 teaspoon vanilla extract
- Mixed berries (such as strawberries, blueberries, raspberries) for topping

Method of Preparation:

1. In a bowl, combine the chia seeds, almond milk, maple syrup (or agave nectar), and vanilla extract.
2. Whisk well to combine all the ingredients.
3. Let the mixture sit for about 5 minutes, then whisk again to break up any clumps.
4. Cover the bowl and refrigerate for at least 2-3 hours, or preferably overnight, to allow the chia seeds to absorb the liquid and thicken.
5. Stir the chia seed pudding before serving to ensure a smooth consistency.
6. Divide the chia seed pudding into serving bowls or glasses.
7. Top with mixed berries.
8. Serve chilled.

Number of Servings: 2

Approximate Caloric Count: Around 200-250 calories per serving

Average Preparation Time: 5 minutes (plus chilling time)

Vegan Banana Bread:

Ingredients:
- 3 ripe bananas
- 1/4 cup coconut oil, melted
- 1/4 cup maple syrup or agave nectar
- 1 teaspoon vanilla extract
- 1 1/2 cups whole wheat flour (or gluten-free flour)
- 1 teaspoon baking soda
- 1/2 teaspoon ground cinnamon
- Pinch of salt
- Optional add-ins: chopped nuts, chocolate chips, dried fruits

Method of Preparation:

1. Preheat the oven to 350°F (175°C). Grease or line a loaf pan with parchment paper.
2. In a large bowl, mash the ripe bananas until smooth.
3. Add the melted coconut oil, maple syrup (or agave nectar), and vanilla extract to the bowl. Stir well to combine.
4. In a separate bowl, whisk together the whole wheat flour, baking soda, ground cinnamon, and salt.
5. Gradually add the dry ingredients to the banana mixture, stirring until just combined. Be careful not to over mix.
6. If desired, fold in any optional add-ins such as chopped nuts, chocolate chips, or dried fruits.
7. Pour the batter into the prepared loaf pan, smoothing the top with a spatula.

8. Bake in the preheated oven for about 50-60 minutes, or until a toothpick inserted into the center comes out clean.
9. Remove the banana bread from the oven and let it cool in the pan for 10-15 minutes before transferring it to a wire rack to cool completely.
10. Slice and serve the vegan banana bread.

Number of Servings: 10-12 slices

Approximate Caloric Count: Around 150-200 calories per serving (slice)

Average Preparation Time: 15-20 minutes (plus baking time)

Apple Cinnamon Crumble:

Ingredients:
- 4 medium apples, peeled, cored, and sliced
- 1 tablespoon lemon juice
- 1/2 teaspoon ground cinnamon
- 1/4 teaspoon ground nutmeg
- 1/4 cup rolled oats
- 1/4 cup whole wheat flour (or gluten-free flour)
- 2 tablespoons coconut sugar (or brown sugar)
- 2 tablespoons coconut oil, melted
- Optional toppings: chopped nuts, coconut flakes, vanilla ice cream (non-dairy)

Method of Preparation:

1. Preheat the oven to 375°F (190°C). Grease a baking dish.
2. In a bowl, combine the sliced apples, lemon juice, ground cinnamon, and ground nutmeg. Toss until the apples are coated.
3. Transfer the apple mixture to the greased baking dish, spreading it out evenly.
4. In another bowl, combine the rolled oats, whole wheat flour, coconut sugar (or brown sugar), and melted coconut oil. Mix well.
5. Sprinkle the crumble mixture evenly over the apples in the baking dish.
6. If desired, sprinkle some chopped nuts or coconut flakes on top for added texture and flavor.

7. Bake in the preheated oven for about 30-35 minutes, or until the apples are tender and the crumble is golden brown.
8. Remove from the oven and let it cool slightly before serving.
9. Serve the apple cinnamon crumble warm, optionally with a scoop of non-dairy vanilla ice cream.

Number of Servings: 4

Approximate Caloric Count: Around 200-250 calories per serving

Average Preparation Time: 15-20 minutes (plus baking time)

Almond Butter Energy Balls:

Ingredients:

- 1 cup rolled oats
- 1/2 cup almond butter (or any nut butter)
- 1/4 cup honey or maple syrup
- 2 tablespoons chia seeds
- 2 tablespoons ground flaxseed
- 1/4 cup dark chocolate chips (or dried fruits, chopped nuts, etc.)
- Pinch of salt

Method of Preparation:

1. In a mixing bowl, combine the rolled oats, almond butter, honey (or maple syrup), chia seeds, ground flaxseed, dark chocolate chips (or other add-ins), and a pinch of salt.
2. Stir well to thoroughly combine all the ingredients.
3. Place the mixture in the refrigerator for about 15-30 minutes to firm up slightly, making it easier to handle.
4. Remove the mixture from the refrigerator and roll it into small balls using your hands. If the mixture is too sticky, wet your hands with water to prevent sticking.
5. Repeat until all the mixture is used, forming energy balls of your desired size.

6. Store the almond butter energy balls in an airtight container in the refrigerator until firm.
7. Serve chilled.

Number of Servings: Makes approximately 12 energy balls

Approximate Caloric Count: Around 100-150 calories per serving (2 energy balls)

Average Preparation Time: 10-15 minutes (plus chilling time)

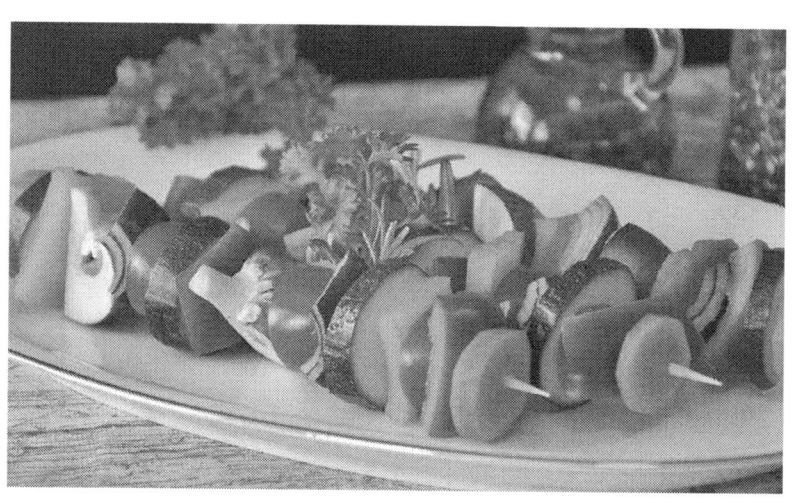

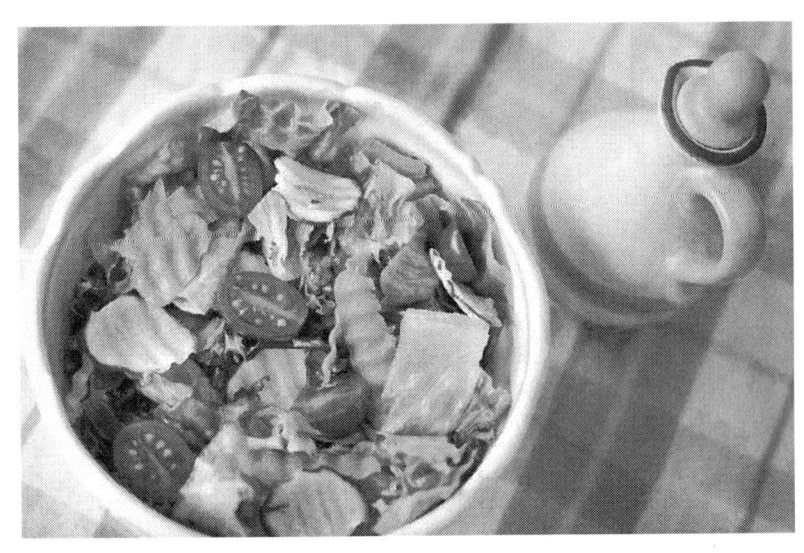

CONCLUSION

As we reach the final pages of this Vegetarian 1200 Calorie Cookbook, we hope that you have been inspired, delighted, and empowered by the recipes and principles shared within. Our journey together has been about more than just creating nutritious and flavorful meals; it's been about embracing a lifestyle that nourishes both your body and soul.

Throughout this book, we have strived to demonstrate that eating a vegetarian diet doesn't mean compromising on taste or satiety. By carefully selecting ingredients and portion sizes, we have crafted a collection of dishes that provide the perfect balance of flavor, nutrition, and calorie control.

By following the 21-day meal plan, you have experienced the benefits of mindful calorie management firsthand. From energizing smoothie bowls in the morning to satisfying main courses and indulgent desserts, you have witnessed the incredible variety and creativity that vegetarian cuisine has to offer. But this is just the beginning.

Beyond the recipes, this book has provided you with a solid foundation for continued success in your journey towards a healthier lifestyle. You have learned about portion control, the importance of balanced nutrition, and the art of mindful eating. Armed with this knowledge, you can now confidently make informed decisions about the foods you consume and the impact they have on your overall well-being.

We encourage you to continue exploring the world of vegetarian cuisine, experimenting with new ingredients, and adapting recipes to suit your taste and dietary needs. Embrace the joy of cooking and sharing meals with loved ones, knowing that you are nourishing your body and supporting a sustainable and compassionate way of life.

As you close this book, remember that the principles and recipes you have discovered here are not confined to these pages. They are a springboard to a lifetime of flavorful, nourishing, and healthful eating. We hope that this Vegetarian 1200 Calorie Cookbook has ignited a passion within you for creating delicious, wholesome meals that bring joy, vitality, and balance to your life.

Thank you for joining us on this culinary journey. May your kitchen be filled with the aromas of delectable dishes and may your plate always be a canvas for both health and indulgence. Here's to a vibrant, delicious, and fulfilling future on your path to vegetarian culinary excellence!

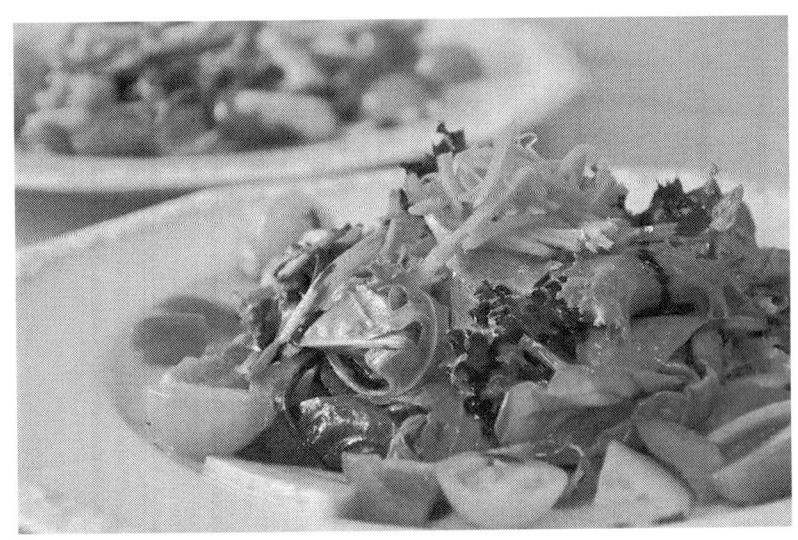

Made in the USA
Monee, IL
31 January 2024